10 BEST

Ways to Manage Stress

KATHLEEN BARNES

TAKE
CHARGE
BOOKS

Brevard, North Carolina

The purpose of this book is to educate. It is not intended for professional medical advice. Any use of the information in this book is at the reader's discretion. This book is sold with the understanding that neither the publisher nor the author has any liability or responsibility for any injury caused or alleged to be caused directly or indirectly by the information contained in this book. While every effort has been made to ensure its accuracy, the book's contents should not be construed as medical advice. To obtain medical advice on your individual health needs, please consult a qualified health care practitioner.

ISBN: 978-0-9883866-0-0

LCCN Number: 2013902883

Cover & interior design by Gary A. Rosenberg
www.thebookcouple.com

Printed in the United States of America

10   9   8   7   6   5   4   3   2   1

Contents

CHAPTER 1   What Is Stress and How Is It Killing You?, 1

CHAPTER 2   Look Out for Number 1, 5

CHAPTER 3   Manage Your Time, 9

CHAPTER 4   Breathe, 13

CHAPTER 5   Meditate, 17

CHAPTER 6   Exercise, 23

CHAPTER 7   Volunteer, 27

CHAPTER 8   Say "No" (and Know When to Say "Yes!"), 31

CHAPTER 9   Build a Community, 35

CHAPTER 10   Embrace Mother Nature, 39

Finally . . . , 42

About the Author, 43

Other Books by Kathleen Barnes, 44

CHAPTER 1

What Is Stress and How Is It Killing You?

If you're alive, you're experiencing stress on a daily basis, perhaps even hourly.

Stress is present in all of our lives. In fact, I venture to say that if you never experience stress, most likely you are dead.

Everywhere we turn, we are challenged. Stress is our response to challenge. It may be something as simple as a minor annoyance when you slosh coffee on your favorite shirt on your way to work to the day-to-day "excitement" that accompanies challenges with kids, spouses, families, bosses, things that don't work, the news cycle and a million other things.

Then there are the stressors most of us recognize: financial worries, job loss, illness, divorce, death.

Even the good stuff is stressful: weddings, births, new jobs, new homes.

Yet stress—at least long-term stress—takes its toll.

Fight or flight

Let's take a brief look at human nature—physical and psychological: Think of our primitive ancestors. Their lives were centered around survival in the midst of an unfriendly world full of challenges. The hunter encountering a hungry saber-toothed tiger or the cavewoman gathering roots who suddenly disturbed a giant anaconda, each instantly developed superhuman powers of combat or escape.

In what is called the "fight or flight" syndrome, when we humans are challenged, we must make an almost instantaneous decision whether to take on the foe or run like hell. Either way, we need to have superior muscle strength at the cost of virtually every other physical process.

In times of fight or flight, digestion comes to a screeching halt. Kidney and liver functions slow to near zero. Everything is focused on keeping the organism alive. That means fleeing or fighting.

The stress hormone adrenaline pumps a surge of energy to muscles, increases blood flow to the extremities and engages brain function so that it is so effective that time seems to slow down and complex thought processes can take place in a split second. This explains how a distraught 120-pound mother can lift a two-ton car off her stricken toddler, a feat of strength normally impossible.

Recovery time

Evolution notwithstanding, our ancestors also learned how to turn off the stress and ratchet down those raging stress hormones once the threat had passed. Once the exhausted hunter reached the safety of his cave or the terrified gatherer found refuge at her hearthfire, the most common response would be to take big drink of water followed by a lengthy period of rest and restoring that innate sense of well-being.

Our ancestors knew how to recover: They took the time to allow the stress response to stop and their bodies to return to normal. The heart rate slowed, digestion and organ function resumes and life was good. They were safe for another day.

Modern day saber-toothed tigers

Now fast forward a few million years to modern times. We are fighting those saber-toothed tigers and giant anacondas day in and day out, years on end, perhaps even for our entire lives.

Of course, these aren't literal saber-toothed tigers and giant anacondas. Instead, it's your son's D in math, your disapproval of your daughter's new boyfriend, the computer that ate the document you need for a key meeting in 15 minutes, a bounced check, the argument with your spouse, the jacket ruined by the dry cleaner, the neighbor's dog that insists on using your yard as his toilet, the guy who cut you off in traffic, nagging worries about the health of an aging parent.

It's life and it's not easy. None of us can escape it.

But the big problem is that we never turn it off. We don't give ourselves a chance to recover, even at the end of a long and stressful day.

We go from that meeting with the cantankerous client to the parent-teacher meeting to whining kids clamoring for dinner to baskets of unfolded laundry, permission slips, tears over math homework, news of war, murder, death and destruction on the television, a dinner of fast food because you're too exhausted to do anything else and getting to bed later than you would like, perhaps lying awake for a couple of hours worrying about an unpaid bill or vague nagging suspicions about your spouse's fidelity, only to have to get up and start all over again five or six hours later.

Forget about exercise. No time.

Stress hormones and their toll on your health

We never stop to let the stress hormones dissipate and allow our bodies to rest and return to their normal function. We just keep pumping adrenaline, noradrenaline and cortisol into our systems until our overloaded systems become ill or even shut down completely.

We get fat because the cortisol glut encourages the buildup of belly fat, the most dangerous kind, increasing the risk of type 2 diabetes and other health problems.

We get heart disease because our overstressed heart muscles can't hold up under years of pumping harder and faster than necessary because of the elevated stress hormones. Blood pressure rises, increasing the risk of heart attack and stroke. It's fair enough to assume that the escape into fast food land has also raised our cholesterol.

We get cancer because the constant presence of stress hormones has damaged us all the way to the cellular level, so our cells no longer are able to reproduce and live and die like normal cells, leading to cancer, Alzheimer's, Parkinson's and more. No wonder the rate of these dread diseases has skyrocketed!

If you have any of these health problems, your chronic stress has become toxic stress. It is dangerous. It is killing you.

In the coming chapters, you'll learn ten simple ways to recognize and manage stress. I won't hedge words: This book will change your life. It may even save your life. Do it and do it now.

CHAPTER 2

Look Out for Number 1

I t might seem like looking out for Number 1 means being selfish. That notion couldn't be farther from the truth.

I was recently on a plane trip and before takeoff, the attendants performed the usual spiel about fastening seatbelts and how to use life vests and oxygen masks. I've heard it a thousand times and you probably have, too. But this time something got my attention. It was the part where they say that you should put your own oxygen mask on first if there is an emergency. No, don't put the mask on your child or your elderly parent first. Why? Because if you pass out from lack of oxygen, who will be there to help them?

Think of it this way: If you're sick, depressed or dysfunctional, how much good are you to your family? Ultimately, if you're no longer around, what good are you to anyone?

Flip back a page or two and review the toll that toxic stress is taking on your health. The truth is plain and simple: If you don't break the stress cycle, you have no future.

If you're a giver and a doer, and you give and give and do and do year in and year out, you're depleting your natural reserves to the point where the reserves will be completely tapped out. Then where will you and your loved ones/coworkers/friends be?

In case you think I might be beating around the bush, I'll tell you plain and simple: You'll be dead and everyone else will be without you.

You *must* put yourself in the Number 1 position in order to discharge those hyperactive stress hormones and to recharge your batteries so you can fight those saber-toothed tigers another day.

I can already hear the excuses why you can't do the things I'm going to recommend in the coming chapters:

"I'm too busy to meditate."

"I don't have time to sit at the beach and sketch."

"Breathe? Ha! If I weren't breathing, I'd be dead."

"I'm too tired to exercise."

"Volunteer? Are you kidding? When would I do that?"

I recognize these excuses because I've made them myself. I also recognize them because they are the hallmarks of someone approaching burnout. They are danger signals. Pay attention.

No compromises on "Me Time"

Start today to carve out some time for yourself every day. Don't let anything get in the way of your "me time." Put it in your calendar and **do not compromise in guarding this time for yourself.**

If that means you must get up earlier, so be it. If it means you need to come straight home from work, speak to no one, lock the bathroom door, draw a bath and spend some time soaking away the day's stresses, do it.

"Me time" means time for you alone. It doesn't count, even if you sit quietly on your deck with your spouse and listen to your favorite music. Why? Because you'll find yourself looking at your spouse, thinking perhaps he looks tired or she has a headache or that the deck needs staining or that the rosebush needs pruning. You'll think of some of those things anyway, but you must do it alone with no thought whatever of anyone or anything else.

I want to tell you about one of the most challenging spiritual practices ever given to me by my teachers. I was to sit for five minutes a day doing absolutely nothing. I was not to meditate, listen to music or do breathing exercises. All of those things are good, but doing nothing was so far outside my box and probably yours, too (or you wouldn't be reading this book) that I found it immensely difficult.

I struggled, squirmed and looked at my watch a dozen times in those interminable five minutes every single day for two months. I argued with myself (and mentally with my spiritual teachers) that I was wasting my time, that I could be doing something more productive, that I was actually increasing my stress levels with this stupid "doing nothing" exercise.

Then one day I felt that resistance let go. It was almost like a rubber band snapped inside me. I finally and blissfully relaxed into the practice. Now I crave those five minutes of doing nothing. I have come to recognize that "doing nothing" is actually doing something profoundly productive. I'm releasing my toxic stress.

You don't have to perform this rigorous exercise, but it is essential that you make Me Time to decompress and de-stress every single day. I won't presume to tell you how much Me Time you need. You will recognize it when you carve out that time. You'll feel your inner rubber band let go.

You might only need that five minutes of doing nothing. You might need an hour of unwinding before bed. Or you might only need 15 minutes with a cup of tea in the morning. You'll also be surprised when you discover that taking those few precious minutes for yourself actually opens up more time in your day because you are more focused and more relaxed as you go about your daily work.

Here are the rules for Me Time:

1. You must do it by yourself.

2. You must do it every day without fail.

3. Me Time cannot involve any type of electronics. This means television, computers, phones in all forms.

4. Enlist the support of your family, if necessary, to respect your Me Time. You may need to work out a swap with your spouse if you have small children who need supervision or wait until they go to sleep.

5. Do not allow any interruptions. Turn off your phone. Don't answer the door.

6. Your Me Time must involve doing something you love.

7. Schedule your Me Time in your calendar. Don't let anything change your appointment with yourself.

8. If your family is open to the idea, you can have everyone have regular Me Time at the same time every day. That can help you avoid interruptions.

9. Schedule more time on weekends if you like, but you cannot diminish the time on weekdays.

10. Vary what you do during your Me Time so that it doesn't become boring or stale.

Only by finding Me Time will you have the energy, patience and self-awareness you need to give to your family, friends, job, and community.

CHAPTER 3

Manage Your Time

Stress is almost always related to time pressure. You've got to hurry to get this or that done, to meet this deadline at work or get the kids to the dentist appointment on time.

Have you ever heard of the Blue Zones? These are a handful of societies on earth where people live exceptionally long lives. They aren't isolated tribes, but live in the modern world and engage in life much like you and me.

But researchers have found a few differences in their lifestyles that extend the average lifespan by 10 or even 20 years. Centenarians are common in these Blue Zones for a variety of reasons, including a largely vegetable based diet, an active lifestyle, close family ties and one key thing to our purpose here: They have stress, but they do not succumb to time pressure. They are not constantly rushing from here to there and spending their lives ratcheting up the stress monster to a level that becomes intolerable, toxic and, ultimately, fatal.

They have learned how to downshift, to take time away from the rat race and refresh themselves. Long-lived Okinawans take time each day to remember their ancestors; Seventh Day Adventists pray; people in Ikaria, Greece, take a nap; and the happy Sardinians have happy hour.

Their secret is finding balance between work and home life, buffers to de-stress in a variety of ways, from spiritual to physical to social. They've found balance in their lives and reaped the rewards of long, healthy lives. Can you say the same?

If your answer is "no," here are some tips that can help you rein the stress that comes from too much to do and never enough time:

- **Plan your day.** A to-do list is an excellent tool to keep you on track. It should include the things you must do and things that you'd like to accomplish. Be realistic and don't overload yourself. You might include something like "make an outline for the first chapter of my new book." Do this every morning. Write it down or program it into your phone. It's very satisfying to check off the tasks you've accomplished. Be sure to include your Me Time.

- **Prioritize.** What is really essential? Many tasks are not really that important but can eat up time like crazy. Take Facebook, for example. I find it very easy to get sucked into the Facebook black hole for an hour and then realize I have to hurry to meet a deadline. Ignore Facebook, set a timer or save it for the end of the day when you can really enjoy it. Ditto for constantly monitoring e-mail or answering every phone call that comes in. Take your To-Do list and assign each entry a 1, 2 or 3 dependent on the urgency of each entry. Do all the 1s first, then the 2s, etc. Also give yourself the leeway not to complete your To-Do list without guilt or extending your workday unreasonably. As an aside: If you're routinely working more than eight hours a day, one of several things may be happening. You may not be working efficiently, there might be unreasonable demands on your time or you have created unnecessary work for yourself. Take some time to reflect on this and decide if you can work smarter, not harder.

- **Don't push the deadline.** Do yourself a huge favor by avoiding last-minute deadline crunches. They are so stressful and they're almost always avoidable. If you have a big project due at work or school or even if you've invited guests and then decided to paint the living room, stay with these projects on a daily basis until they're done. When you were in school, did you pull all-nighters before finals? Most of us probably did and most of us regretted it. If you did, you know you felt exhausted for days afterward and that last-minute studying probably didn't improve your grade. It might have even hurt your grade.

- **Eat the elephant one bite at a time.** How do you eat an elephant? One bite at a time! This goes right along with not pushing the deadline. It's easy to get overwhelmed when there is a huge task at hand. What comes next? You throw in the towel and avoid it altogether or get yourself so stressed that you have a melt-down. Say you have to clean out the house of a deceased relative or you suffered temporary insanity and agreed to organize the library at your child's school or coordinate a planning team at work that will launch a new spinoff company. All of these tasks are daunting, but they are all doable if you break them up in bite-sized pieces. Start with a list of all the tasks that must be completed and in what order. Now (this is extremely important) make a list of people who might help you, including volunteer help and hired help. Next, schedule out the timeframe, or if there is not a specific deadline, give yourself a deadline so it doesn't drag out forever. Now estimate the time it will take to complete the task, which will give you an idea of how much time you need to devote to the project on a daily or weekly or monthly basis.

- **Follow the 10-minute rule.** So you hate cleaning the bathroom? Filing away paperwork? Writing your monthly work report at work? Doing your daily strength training? This one is sort of like eating the elephant, too, but it may involve a task that really isn't that big, but it's one you really dislike. So grit your teeth and do it anyway, but just for 10 minutes at a time. Most of us can tolerate anything for 10 minutes, so go for it. You might even decide you like the task over time. If not and it is something you must do (pare down that list of MUSTs to the bare mini-mum), soldier on for the 10 minutes at a pop and you won't burn out.

- **De-clutter.** Whether it is on your desk or in your closet or garage, nearly all of us have too much stuff. I believe that excess "stuff" is energetically draining, since we are emotionally and sometimes physically attached to it. If getting rid of stuff is dis-tasteful, use the 10-minute rule. Generally you can clean out a drawer or put away a few files in 10 minutes. Someone once told me to look around my house and unless I could honestly say that I *loved* everything there (not just "liked" the stuff), out it went. The result is amazingly freeing and there is so much less to clean. I mean, do you really need the shirt you wore for your seventh-grade class photo? Create a goal to have at least one empty drawer in each room and keep it that way.

- **Take a break.** We humans are hard wired to multitask. Nothing spells burnout faster than driving the same widget into the same frame on an assembly line all day long or sitting in front of a computer or even teaching back-to-back-to-back Pilates classes. I spend much of my time in front of my computer screen. It's not surprising that my brain gets foggy and my body gets stiff from inactivity. So I take an activity break. It's great for me to do some fairly mindless repetitive activity, so I'll go out in the gar-den and pull weeds for 15 minutes or do a little yoga or take a short brisk walk or even file some of those dread papers. They all help me refocus and, far from goofing off, they help me to work more efficiently and be more productive. If you have a very physical job, say in construction or teaching those Pilates classes, you can rest your body and brain by sitting down and putting up your feet for a few minutes, perhaps stimulating your brain with a crossword puzzle or a newsmagazine or some med-itative music.

CHAPTER 4

Breathe

Breath is life. Quite literally without breath, life ends in just a few minutes.

Some Eastern traditions believe that we are born with a finite numbers of breaths allotted to us, so the more deeply and slowly we breathe, the longer we will live.

Here's something to think about: Imagine you are driving your car and another car drifts over into your lane. You sound your horn and perhaps make a hand gesture or two toward the other driver. It's a near-miss and there is no accident and no one is injured.

What's happening to you? Not only are you perhaps uttering a few choice words, your heart is pounding, your senses are hyper-alert—and your breath is shallow and fast.

If you stop your car, sit still and take ten deep breaths, everything changes in short order. Your heart rate returns to normal, the hyper-awareness and energy rush dissipate and everything mellows out.

Of course, what I'm describing here is a typical stress challenge and release. Remembering that we talked about unrelieved and toxic stress and our inability to release it in Chapter 1, you'll see how powerful those few deep breaths can be to help you release the stress.

I'll start with the most basic deep breathing. This may be all you need, but there are other types of breath you can employ for different levels of stress.

Basic deep breathing

Let's start with some basic physiology. I promise it will be painless.

Your lungs are the size of two footballs. They can hold a large volume of air, yet most of us use only about the upper one-third of our lung capacity. The diaphragm is a membrane that stretches across your torso beneath your lungs, and when your belly is relaxed, the diaphragm allows your lungs to inflate fully.

It is natural to relax the belly for maximum lung capacity when you inhale and to contract the belly when you exhale. All of us breathe this way when we are asleep. Children and animals breathe this way. Somewhere along the line, most of us somehow got switched. I attribute it to the old Mom admonition to "Stand up straight, put your shoulders back and suck your belly in." This time, Mom was wrong.

Deep belly breathing fills your body with oxygen and helps expel waste products most efficiently through the carbon dioxide exchange in the lungs.

To practice basic deep breathing, sit comfortably with your spine straight and your shoulders relaxed. At the beginning, it helps to put your hands on your belly so you can get a better sense of its movement.

Now take in a deep slow breath through your nose. Feel your belly push slightly against your hands as you fill your lungs completely. As soon as your lungs are as full as you can comfortably inhale, immediately begin to exhale, again, slowly and comfortably, slightly contracting your abdominal muscles to help expel all the air.

Continue breathing this way for several minutes. If this type of breathing is new to you, you may begin to feel a little light-headed. That is simply because your system is not accustomed to so much oxygen. The light-headed feeling will pass. If it is too uncomfortable, keep your breath slightly more shallow until your body adjusts.

Here are several other breathing techniques that will help you relieve stress:

1. **Ocean breath.** Yogis call this breath "ujjaya." It's the basic breathing technique with an added element: You make the sound of the ocean in the base of your throat. Imagine you are breathing in at that point at the base of your throat. This results in a slight vibration there that sounds almost like you are beginning to snore. When your inhalation is complete, exhale using the same sound, contracting your abdominal muscles as you squeeze out the breath. The added sounds increase your relaxation and give you a focal point for some meditation techniques, as we will discuss in Chapter 5.

2. **Holding breath.** The holding breath is an extension of the basic breath with the added element of holding briefly after the inhalation. Dr. Andrew Weil teaches a balancing breath that I love:

   • Inhale for the count of eight.

   • Hold for the count of seven.

   • Exhale for the count of eight.

   • Repeat four times.

   • Very simple and very effective for stress relief!

3. **Breathe into the pain.** You have no doubt discovered that stress can result in physical pain, most often from tight muscles. Using the basic breath, mentally focus the breath into the sore area. For instance, if your neck is sore, mentally send the breath and the relief to your neck to relax those tight muscles. Ditto for a shoulder, back and even belly pain.

4. **Cooling breath.** If you're feeling hot (physically or emotionally), the cooling breath will cool you off quickly. Being mindful of the basic breathing technique, breathe in normally and exhale through pursed lips as though you are blowing gently through a straw. Repeat 8 to 10 times for a fast cool-off.

5. **Emergency breath**. Okay, so you've avoided the car accident, the confrontation with your spouse or your child's insolence, but you just can't seem to let go of it. You're replaying the situation over and over in your head. Start with the basic breath for a minute or two and then add the emergency bailout:

- The best position is sitting on your heels on the floor with your hands on the floor in front of you. If you can't do that, sit in a chair, feet flat on the floor with your hand on the edge of a sturdy table in front of you.

- Straightening your arms, take a vigorous breath in through your nose.

- Immediately exhale vigorously through your nose as you bend your arms.

- Do 8 to 10 breaths this way. You can repeat for a second round if you wish.

This is a powerful and intense technique. It will almost certainly make you feel light-headed, so take it easy and be sure not to get up too quickly when you finish.

CHAPTER 5

Meditate

Meditation isn't complicated or particularly esoteric. Your Me Time and your breathing exercises are a great preparation time for meditation because it is teaching you to be still and to break the stress cycle.

Really, that's all that meditation is: Stilling the mind. Since we know the mind and body and spirit are all interwoven, stilling the mind will heal body and spirit as well.

Meditation has been practiced for thousands of years, but modern science is just catching on to the ancient truth: Meditation can change your body as well as your mind. Dozens of scientific studies show the physiological benefits of meditation. Research suggests that meditation may help with:

- allergies
- anxiety disorders
- asthma
- binge eating
- cancer
- depression

- fatigue
- heart disease
- high blood pressure
- pain
- sleep problems
- substance abuse

You don't have to meditate for hours on end—10 or 15 minutes daily should suffice.

There are many forms of meditation. I'm going to introduce you to just a few here. Some may be more effective for you than others, so it's a good idea to try out more than one.

The basics

Meditation should not become a chore or a duty. It takes about three weeks to form a new habit. I promise if you faithfully practice daily meditation for three weeks, this stress-relieving habit will be - come a part of your consciousness and your daily practice will become a joy that you eagerly anticipate.

If you make that three-week commitment, the rest is a piece of cake!

What follows is the most elementary description of the most commonly used meditation techniques. This is an incredibly complex subject that merits far greater depth. I cover these individual techniques in greater depth in my book *10 Best Ways to Meditate*.

For most forms of sitting meditation, you should sit in a chair or on the floor with your spine straight and your feet flat on the floor. It's best not to lie down because that's the position most of us assume for sleeping and our subconscious minds are programmed to connect lying down with going to sleep. Many meditators like to have their hands resting comfortably, palms up on their knees with thumbs and forefingers in circles to contain energy.

I like to use a particular shawl that I've had for more than 20 years for practical reasons because body temperatures tend to drop as we become relaxed and for spiritual reasons because this shawl contains the energy of many, many years of meditation. Also, the act of putting on the shawl places my mind in readiness to let go of distraction and for my body to let go of stress.

Now, relax your shoulders.

Turn off your phone and eliminate distractions as much as possible. You may find that some soft soothing music will be helpful. Earbuds can help block out external distractions.

10 BEST MEDITATIONS

1. **Guided visualization.** This is perhaps the easiest form of meditation for beginners because you will have a teacher whose voice leads you into the meditation and perhaps introduces you to a peaceful place or even in search of guides or power animals. These types of meditations are available everywhere as MP3 downloads, on CDs and even on You Tube. Look for my name—Kathleen Barnes—on YouTube for a very short guided imagery meditation and, if you like it, download one of several full guided imagery journeys from my website: www.kathleenbarnes.com/meditation.

2. **Follow the breath.** Simply follow your breath in and out, relaxing your belly as you breathe in and contracting it slightly as you breathe out. Keep your focus on your breath. If you become distracted, think of the thoughts running through your mind as clouds passing by a beautiful blue sky and gently bring yourself back to the breath. The essence of this form of meditation is in understanding that for this small space in time, there is nothing to do or think except to follow the breath.

3. **Progressive relaxation.** This is one type of meditation that you might find is more effective if you are lying down. Starting with your feet, tense, hold and relax every muscle group. For example, point your toes away from your head and then toward your head, hold a few seconds and release. Progressing upward to and including your scalp, this technique releases deeply held stress patterns in every part of your body.

4. **Floating meditation.** This one is particularly effective for you water babies. Imagine yourself floating in an endless ocean that is the perfect temperature, warm and welcoming. The waves gently rock you up and down. You are completely safe and secure in the arms of this great ocean. Music that features the sounds of the ocean can help get you to this place of relaxation.

5. **Candle meditation.** If you have some difficulty keeping your eyes closed, try putting a lighted candle about three feet in front of you and darkening the rest of the room as much a possible. Simply focus your attention on the candle until your eyes begin to close involuntarily. This means you have reached a state of meditation.

6. **Mantra meditation.** A mantra is a word or chant repeated out loud over and over, quieting the mind and releasing stress. From the basic sitting position, simply repeat your mantra over and over. You can experiment with different mantras. You may have experienced the mantra "Om," the universal sound of inner peace. You can also use "One" or "I am" or "Peace." You can use almost any words that calm your mind. Get creative!

7. **Chakra meditation.** Chakras are the body's energy centers. Most experts agree there are at least seven, perhaps many more. The chakras are aligned from the base of the spine to the top of the head in a specific order and are associated with specific colors, emotions and sexuality:

   • Red: basic security, physical well-being; the base of the spine

   • Orange: sexuality; just below the belly button

   • Yellow: intellect, power; solar plexus

   • Green: love, healing; heart

   • Blue: feelings and communicating feelings; throat

   • Purple: spiritual truths; third eye center between the eyebrows

   • White: enlightenment; crown of the head

   Simply visualize these colors at these particular body points from the bottom to the top.

8. **Moving meditation.** This can involve walking or spontaneous movement. It is ideal for those who have trouble sitting still for

extended periods of time. The difference here from ordinary walking or exercising is that it is done very slowly (you might cover 100 feet in a 10-minute walking meditation) and with complete attention to the movement, focusing inward and to the point of stillness. Some forms of yoga, including the Kripalu yoga that I teach, employ conscious and spontaneous movement as a form of meditation.

9. **Mindfulness meditation.** Continually focus your mind on the present, gently returning your focus to the present each time your thoughts wander. This is one of the mostly commonly practiced Buddhist meditation techniques based on the premise that there is no moment except the present, the Now.

10. **Spiritual meditation.** This is a misnomer, since all meditation is spiritual, but this form is interchangeable with what most of us think of as prayer. The process involves clearing your mind by deeply breathing and intentional focus, then posing a question and waiting in stillness for an answer.

In conclusion, these techniques all take some time to learn. Try the various basic techniques and you will likely find one that really works for you. Everyone is different and for a wide variety of reasons, some techniques will work more easily for you than others. That is all as it should be.

It is very important that you do not beat yourself up if you have difficulty. The human mind is very strong and is ultraconservative, not in the political sense, but in the physiological sense that it fights like crazy to preserve the status quo. The mind resists change, even if the present is very uncomfortable.

So expect some pushback from your mind. Persist and you will succeed.

Again, I cover all of these techniques in greater depth in my book *10 Best Ways to Meditate*.

CHAPTER 6

Exercise

Here's the secret of exercise:
You've got to love it.

I mean you have to love what you're doing, or quite simply, you won't do it. That's why so many people join gyms or buy treadmills and make these great New Year's resolutions in January that are abandoned by March.

If you love tennis, by all means, play tennis, daily, if possible. If you are a loner who wants to walk in the woods alone, that's your answer. Maybe it's playing pickup volleyball on the beach or taking a Zumba class. Don't try to swim against the river here. Your basic form of exercise *must* be something you truly enjoy.

Exercise can become an addiction and a very positive one for stress relief. Exercise causes your brain to release substances called endorphins, which are natural feel-good brain chemicals and pain relievers. Quite simply, that makes you want more.

Moving your body is one of the most powerful stress relievers known, according to the prestigious Mayo Clinic. Better yet, any type of movement will result in stress relief, so I prefer to call it movement therapy rather than exercise. It seems more digestible.

Movement will also help relieve depression and anxiety, as I cover in depth in my book *10 Best Ways to Beat Depression.*

You don't know what kind of exercise you love? Maybe you actually hate exercise. About one-third of Americans do no conscious exercise at all, to their detriment. I don't think it is an accident that this is in the ballpark of the numbers who report they are chronically depressed. The two go very much hand in hand, but that's a subject to be explored in depth in my depression book.

I can understand the resistance to exercise. Many people have that affliction. In fact, I can also understand how stress-producing it might be to hear me tell you that you need to add an hour of exercise a day to your already maxed-out stressful lifestyle. It's not going to happen, is it?

How about we take it in little bites?

- Can you manage a 10-minute walk a day? Maybe on your lunch break?

- Can you walk up the stairs to your office or appointment?

- How about parking at the far end of the row when you shop?

You can actually get in a surprising amount of movement therapy in these small bites. In fact, researchers at Arizona State University found that three 10-minute walks a day reduced blood pressure more than one 30-minute walk.

So if three walks sounds too hard, try just one.

Walking

I'm not going to pretend to be able to tell you what is the best form of exercise for you. In fact, I choose to think of a lifetime of movement rather than so much conscious exercise.

Here's what I do:

I'm a walking addict. Bear with me, even if this isn't your passion. Walking is the easiest, most universal, cheapest way to get movement therapy. You can quite literally do it any time, any place. All you need is a comfortable pair of shoes. Period. You don't need any memberships. You don't need a buddy, although it is nice to have one sometimes. Generally, you don't get sweaty and need to changes clothes and shower.

I do it rain or shine, 7 days a week *because I love it*. I'm lucky enough to live in the mountains and our neighborhood has lots of trails and friendly neighbors who don't mind respectful walkers on their land. After my 100-pound weight-loss program, I decided walking would be my forever friend. I bought a pedometer, wear it every day and aim for 10,000 steps a day. I make it most days, and occasionally go way over, usually if I'm involved in a gardening binge and lose myself in the work, not even thinking about the "exercise" side of it.

Just as an aside, movement therapy or exercise doesn't have to be what most people think. Gardening is a powerful form of exercise that involves all the muscle groups. What's more, we tend to sustain it longer because we're focused on the task at hand, weeding a bed, planting some new flowers or harvesting vegetables. Gardening is stress relieving in many ways, partly because you're making a grounding connection with the Earth by putting your hands in the soil and clearing out unneeded clutter in the form of weeds. It's not hard at all to burn 400 calories an hour while gardening. That's more than jogging. Hey, even vacuuming and grocery shopping keep you moving. I like to stand up and work on my laptop from time to time, too. That's the whole idea: Just move it!

I love my walking time. It's a meditation for me, too, and being out in nature fills me with peace. That's a huge stress reliever for me.

If I'm grappling with a question, dilemma, how to write something or how to address a difficult situation with someone, I can find answers when I "switch gears" and take a walk.

Yes, I admit it. I'm addicted.

Exercise improves coping skills

There's also something about exercise that helps the body cope better with stress, according to the American Psychological Association. At least one study suggests that the brain chemical norepinephrine may also be enhanced by exercise, enabling the brain to deal more efficiently with stress. The same paper suggests that exercise gives the body a chance to practice dealing with stress, enabling better communication among the various body systems that are part of the stress response.

In a way, you're actually exercising your body's ability to respond to stress. There are some theories that say exercise actually increases your body's ability to cope with long-term stress, the kind of stress I call toxic stress.

Exercise saves time

We're all time-stressed and most of us think we haven't got a spare moment even to add those few minutes of daily exercise.

The truth is you can't afford *not* to take that time. Exercise actually is key to better focus and an ability to work in a more focused and productive way.

Exercise also helps erase the cobwebs and brain fog that frequently accompany stressful times. Think about it: You're sitting at your desk with a dozen files open in front of you and a deadline looming. What to do? You are in a complete dither and you feel your blood pressure rising.

Stop. Take a few breaths. Push yourself back from your desk and go for a brisk 10-minute walk. That's all it takes and you're back at your desk, brain fog gone. That's because you've simply increased the flow of oxygen and glucose (the brain's food) through the bloodstream, reenergizing you exactly when you need it.

Mayo Clinic also suggests that exercise helps you get focused and erase background irritations and frustrations so you can concentrate on the task at hand, stressful or not.

In conclusion, exercise is your easiest, cheapest, most accessible stress reliever. There's nothing more to it than to walk out your door. We all know how to do it and there are no special techniques. Unless you are severely disabled, you can most likely take a 10-minute walk here and there. Don't worry about technique. Don't worry about anything. Just go for it.

In addition, exercise improves sleep quality, and we all know that things tend to look different in the morning after a good night's sleep.

CHAPTER 7

Volunteer

So I'm asking you to commit to *more* time? That doesn't make sense, you're probably saying.

Actually, it makes perfect sense. Here's why:

Doing something for someone else always shifts your focus from yourself to something about which you care passionately.

Most people think they have not a spare moment for anything else in their already stress-filled lives, but they find that paying it forward (like in the movie of the same name) actually reaps rewards in terms of increased relaxation, less anxiety and less time pressure.

There's a zen of chopping veggies at the local soup kitchen a couple of hours a week or walking dogs for your incapacitated neighbor or reading to kids in a day-care center.

There's also the good feeling of doing something for someone who is appreciative of your efforts and of sharing your energies with someone who needs help.

"Yes, but . . ." I hear you say. "There's still the time issue."

Can you cut out some activities that are not as important to put in a small commitment that impassions you? The rewards will make it well worthwhile. Is it really necessary to fully clean your house each week? Will a lick and a promise do the trick? Maybe you could give up an hour or two of Facebook time. . . .

Can you combine a couple of stress relievers, for example exercise and volunteerism, such as a local walk-a-thon for a cause that is dear to you or joining a meditation group for world peace? (As we all know, peace begins within each of us.)

Studies show that doing good for others is good for your emotional well-being and can measurably enhance your peace of mind. One study found that dialysis patients, transplant patients and family members who volunteered to help other patients experienced increased personal growth and emotional well-being. Another study on patients with multiple sclerosis showed that those who offered other MS patients support actually reported greater benefits than the patients they helped, including more pronounced improvement on confidence, self-awareness, self-esteem, depression and daily functioning. Those who volunteered almost universally found their lives changed dramatically and positively with far less stress.

What goes around comes around

I'm a firm believer in the law of karma, which says you get back what you give and then some, for good or for bad.

In simple terms, if you are a taker who constantly demands from others without giving back, you'll eventually get taken, probably in a most unpleasant way. If you abuse your spouse or children, you will be abused in one way or another.

Karma does not always come back to you from the place it was incurred. If you kick the dog, it doesn't necessarily mean he'll bite you, but he might.

On the converse side of negative karma, you reap the good you give.

What goes around comes around. You get more than you give when you volunteer and, like in some of the exercise studies, volunteering increases resilience in times of stress.

When we make selfless personal sacrifices, we reap what we sow in the form of favors from others. People known as "givers" universally receive all manner of positive benefits, usually not from those they helped or even those connected with the places they helped. The returns and the social support you earn through giving to others, combined with the good feelings you get from helping others more than make up for the sacrifices you make to offer your assistance.

So, this is a simple one: Give and you will receive. Your stress will decrease, your life will improve and everything around you will change.

CHAPTER 8

Say "No"
(and Know When
to Say "Yes!")

This chapter very intentionally follows the chapter on the stress-relief benefits of volunteering and saying a resounding "yes."

I think it was Judith Orloff who said, " 'No' is a one-word sentence."

Wow! That one really hit me hard. On the rare occasions I say "no," the answer is usually accompanied by a long explanation about how busy I am, why I can't coordinate the PTA bake sale, etc. Let's be straightforward about it—I say "no" because I don't want to do whatever is being requested of me.

Now, I am in my 60s and have proudly achieved full cronehood. That means I have every right to say "no" for whatever reason I want and anytime I want. I don't owe anyone an expla nation.

I don't have to be impolite. I can say, "No, but thanks for thinking of me." I can smile and even suggest someone else who might take on whatever task is being requested, but the answer is still firmly "no."

Degrees of "Yes"

The lesson of "No is a one-word sentence" goes hand in hand with another lesson I learned somewhere about the shadings of "yes."

It goes something like this:

Your friend asks, "Would you like to go see the new Brad Pitt movie?"

I might immediately reply, very enthusiastically, "Yes!"

That is the only genuine "yes." All other wishy-washy forms of "yes" are really "no."

When my friend asks about the Brad Pitt movie and I respond, "Well, maybe . . ." or "Maybe next week" to be polite, the answer is really "no." I can let her know I'd like to spend time with her, but I'm not really interested in that movie or I'd really rather curl up at home with a book tonight or I have scheduled Me Time or whatever. You'll know right in your gut if it is a "YES!" Everything else is "no."

The power of "no" is that we marshall our time and don't let extraneous and unwanted activities become stressors. It also nurtures self-esteem when we are able to be truthful, but not brutal. Finally, saying "no" empowers us to choose the things we want and love to do rather than trying to meet the expectations of others.

Don't be a doormat

I know someone who will remain anonymous because she is a dearly loved family member, who was constantly imposed upon by her in-laws. They treated her as a cook (she's an excellent one) and maid and expected her to create weekly gourmet feasts to which they contributed nothing in terms of money or energy.

In addition to having a full-time job, being a full-time student and having two young children, she was overwhelmed by this expectation. I call it an inconsiderate imposition. I'd like to say that she was able to empower herself with "no," but the reality was that she was afraid of losing their love and esteem. She had to suffer a fairly serious health crisis before the in-laws realized for themselves that they were asking too much. The matter resolved itself when she moved two hours away from the leeching in-laws and her kitchen was no longer an easy drop-in café.

She had become a doormat and didn't know how to extract herself.

Learning to say "No"

If you won't protect yourself, who will?

When was the last time you said "no"?

Maybe it would be even more revealing if I ask you, when was the last time you said "YES!"?

It may be hard to stick up for yourself and call people when they impose on your good will or to let people know that now is not the time for you to commit time to their pet project or that you simply aren't interested.

Sometimes it's hard to be polite in the face of a hard sell and sometimes you have to really dig in your feet.

I have a particular friend who has a passion for clogging, an Appalachian form of dance. She is very passionate about it and spends a significant number of hours a week promoting her clogging club, creating costumes, raising money for them and going to competitions. Her passion for clogging is infectious. She is dogged in her determination to get me to come along with her, but my interest level is zero to none. It's just not my thing. I have told her that on several occasions, but it didn't deter her. Eventually I realized that I had begun avoiding her phone calls because I didn't want to hear another sales pitch about clogging.

I was finally able to convince her to stop badgering me about clogging when I reflected back to her the fact that she does not share my interest in my spiritual path. That somehow struck home, and we were able to resume our friendship and stop the pressure.

We all think we know what might be best for someone else, but the truth is you only know what is in your own heart, and if you take some time to look at it, you'll know what is right for you, too.

One more story comes to mind, which I thought was a fairly creative (and truthful) way to say "no" without being harsh.

My local political party committee wanted me to accept a countywide office. They think I am a pretty organized person, which I am, but they didn't have a clue about the depth of my dislike for that kind of job. I would rather sleep on a bed of nails or have a root canal than to take a job like that. My first, second and third thoughts were a resounding "NO!"

But I didn't want to be rude. There is no percentage in that.

So what did I tell them? I smiled and said that I was too opinionated. I could not tow the party line and work for candidates that I didn't approve of or smile and be nice when I really wanted to throttle some of the elected officials. Did it work? Like a charm! They haven't asked again, nor are they likely to.

CHAPTER 9

Build a Community

Have you ever had a bitch buddy?

I can remember a particularly stressful period of my life when I had lots of complaints. I had a friend who was going through something similar, so we agreed to allow each other three minutes a day of phone time unmitigated bitching. We'd give each other a sympathetic ear with the occasional interruption for a neutral "Mmhmmm" or "Poor you."

Part of our agreement was we didn't try to counsel each other or "fix" anything. We just listened. And we did each other an enormous favor by simply allowing each other to have a non-judgmental outlet for the stresses of the day.

After three minutes each (and, yes, we'd time it), time was up and we'd move on to more positive conversation or simply thank each other and hang up.

Maggie and I were bitch buddies for a few months and the need dissolved. We remained friends, and although we now live far apart and we've drifted apart over the years, I am eternally grateful for her sympathetic ear when I really needed it.

Create community

We need each other. Whether it is a loving spouse to rub your shoulders at the end of a tough day or a child who offers to cook dinner (no matter how "interesting" it might be!) or your mom, sister, bitch buddy, walking partner or neighbor, we create our "communities" to fulfill our needs.

Countless studies show that people with a balanced, happy social support structure experience fewer stress-related physiological symptoms and are better stress managers than people without social support. Your loved ones are also in an excellent position to observe your lifestyle and offer suggestions and help when you need it.

If you already have a social support network, use it. If you don't, create one.

"Oh yeah," I hear you grumble. "And when will I have time to do *that*?"

My answer: Find the time. Make the time, even though hyperstress tends to make you want to go into a shell. Do it. It is that important. Spend that six minutes on the phone with your bitch buddy. Remember payback: you have to listen to his or her complaints, too! Take a 15-minute walk with your spouse after dinner. You can get in three stress relievers at once this way: exercise, time in nature and community. Have a cup of coffee with your best friend. It will make a huge difference in your ability to cope with the stressors of your day.

You'll notice the title of this chapter is "Build a Community." Your support network doesn't happen all by itself. It is an investment of time, energy and love. Remember this is a pay-it-forward situation. You will find your support network evaporates if you are constantly asking for help and never giving back. Be there for your friends when you are needed and you'll reap lifelong friendships.

Other kinds of togetherness

1. **Make a date with your mate.** If sex has been on the bottom of your to-do list for too long, move it to the top. Sex increases levels of endorphins, those mood-boosting chemicals in the brain and it's one of the best total-body relaxers around. If necessary,

put it on both of your calendars and don't let anything get in the way. No partner? Well, you know there is such a thing as DIY.

2. **Get a pet.** Numerous studies show that pets help lower blood pressure. Just having a cat sit on your lap or petting a dog has a tremendous calming effect. If you don't have a pet, consider getting one. You'll find a friend for life at your local animal shelter. Rescue is my favorite breed. If for some reason you absolutely cannot have a pet, visit a friend's menagerie regularly.

3. **Join a church or spiritual group.** Studies also show very emphatically that those who take time for spirituality at least once a week (more is better, in my opinion) are more relaxed, have fewer illnesses and actually live longer.

CHAPTER 10

Embrace Mother Nature

We are meant to be in sync with the rhythms of the earth. Our ancestors lived by the sun and moon and their lives were centered around the changing of the seasons.

We modern-day humans spend most of our lives indoors, fixated on flickering computer and television screens and then we wonder why we feel disconnected.

A friend who has taught recovery programs for alcoholics and drug abusers for more than 20 years recently told me she thought the source of all addiction is separation from our natural connection with the Earth. That turned on a light for me.

I would add to her theory that the source of unrelieved stress is also our disconnection from our natural place in the universe.

Who can feel stressed walking on a beach or working in a garden or hiking in the mountains?

Mother Nature truly is our mother. We can give her everything that bothers us and she accepts it without judgment.

I remember a time several years ago, when I was going through a great deal of stress. I can tell you that it was so long ago that we were still using incandescent light bulbs, because the stress levels and unfocussed energy were actually giving off enough electromagnetic energy that I was blowing out light bulbs on nearly a daily basis. I joked that I should buy stock in a light-bulb manufacturer, but it really wasn't funny. When my unresolved stress energy blew out my computer monitor, I realized that the next step might be to blow out some circuit in my body, so I sent out a wide appeal for help to friends and colleagues.

You'd think as a yoga teacher for 25 years at the time I would have had the tools to resolve my own overstressed situation, but I didn't. In fact, I've noticed over the years for myself and those I have coached, when the going gets rough, we tend to forget all the tools at hand.

When the answers came back, there were two that jumped out at me.

The first, from a friend who was always right but never gentle: "Get your butt out to your garden. Get your hands in the dirt. Let the stress drain off into the Earth. Pull some weeds and plant something new."

And from a spiritual advisor: "Get a stone about the size of a basketball. Put it outside your front door and designate it as your grounding stone. Go outside and put your hands on it when you feel your stress levels mounting."

I followed both pieces of advice, since they were somewhat similar and I never blew out another light bulb. I still work in my garden daily in spring, summer and fall and weekly even in winter. It grounds me and gives me great peace and joy.

Interestingly, my grounding stone appeared just a few days after I was instructed to find one: It's a large piece of turquoise (yes, almost the size of a basketball) brought from Arizona by some wandering friends who thought I'd like it. It's still outside my front door, and I still use it regularly when I feel the stress building up.

Mother Nature invites us to slow down. She is rarely rushed and she offers good advice there.

1. **Take that walk during your lunch hour.** Stroll along and notice trees, flowers, birds and clouds.

2. **Find a time to be outside** and in nature for at least 15 minutes every day.

3. **Look out the window** if you can't get outside for some reason. Appreciate the beauty of nature.

4. **Put on your headphones** and chill out to the sounds of nature on one of the many places you can find them online. The sounds of rain, ocean waves, the rain forest and more will transport you away from stress and help you release and relax.

5. **Find some beautiful nature pictures for your screensaver.** You'll definitely get the feeling looking at a picture of a serene beach or a majestic mountain view.

6. **Put a birdfeeder outside your window** and invite the winged ones to join you.

7. **Bring nature inside,** even if you are able to spend quite a bit of time outdoors. Fill your house with plants, stones, shells, crystals and feathers. They'll all renew your connection with nature every time you touch them.

8. **Set up an indoor fountain.** The sound of splashing water is an instant stress reliever.

Finally...

I hope this book has given you some insight into the nature of stress and offered some concrete ways to relieve stress.

The next step: Prevent chronic stress in the first place. You know what it looks like. You know its effects on your life and your health. Now you have the tools. Go for it!

About the Author

Kathleen Barnes is a passionate natural health advocate, author, writer and publisher who has devoted more than 30 years to educating the public about healthy living. She is an unusually versatile writer with more than 40 years of experience as a journalist in print, broadcast and online media and as an author, editor and publisher with 14 books to her credit, most of them on natural health subjects.

Kathleen's passion for natural health and sustainable living has its roots in the early days of the natural health movement.

She has coached clients through health, career and relationship transformations for more than three decades. She is also a certified Kripalu Yoga teacher.

Contact Kathleen through her website: www.kathleenbarnes.com.

She would love to hear from you, your experiences, suggestions for new titles and other feedback. She also invites you to leave a review of this book on Amazon.com.

OTHER BOOKS BY KATHLEEN BARNES

10 Best Ways to Meditate (Take Charge Books, 2013)

10 Best Ways to Manage Depression (Take Charge Books 2013)

The Super Simple HCG Diet (Square One Publishing, 2011)

Rx from the Garden: 101 Food Cures You Can Easily Grow (Adams Media, 2011)

The Calcium Lie: What Your Doctor Doesn't Know Could Kill You with Dr. Robert Thompson (In Truth Press, 2008)

8 Weeks to Vibrant Health: A Take Charge Plan for Women with Dr. Hyla Cass (first edition McGraw-Hill, 2005, second edition, Take Charge Books, 2008)

The Secret of Health: Breast Wisdom with Dr. Ben Johnson (Morgan James, 2008)

User's Guide to Hypothyroidism (Basic Health Publications, 2006)

Users Guide to Natural Menopause (Basic Health Publications, 2005)

Arthritis and Joint Health (Woodland Publishing, 2005)

Coming Soon:

Let the Sun Shine In: The Miracle of Vitamin D

10 Best Breathing Techniques

10 Best Ways to Prevent Memory Loss, Alzheimer's and Dementia

10 Best Ways to Care for Someone with Alzheimer's or Dementia

www.ingramcontent.com/pod-product-compliance
Lightning Source LLC
Chambersburg PA
CBHW060626030426
42337CB00018B/3227